How to Lose Thigh Fat

I0438422

The Most Effective and Simple Solutions to Trim your Thighs

Allison Lewis

Table of Contents

Introduction

I want to thank you and congratulate you for purchasing the book, "*How to Lose Thigh Fat: The Most Effective and Simple Solutions to Trim your Thighs*".

This book contains proven steps and strategies on how to successfully lose those unwanted fats in your thighs by simply improving your diet and getting more physical activity into your lifestyle.

Trying to lose your thigh fat is an almost impossible goal to achieve. However, getting yourself to commit to eating well, following a healthy weight-loss diet plan, keeping your body fit with regular exercise, and performing thigh-targeted workout routines will go a long way when it comes to pushing yourself to have thinner thighs more quickly.

This book provides you plenty of easy-to-follow tips that only require your determination and patience. You absolutely do not need any special gym equipment or food supplements to practice all the helpful information offered by this book.

Thanks again for purchasing this book, I hope you enjoy it!

Chapter 1 - Practice Healthy Eating

Losing fat in your thighs requires you to lose the overall excess fat in your body, and to be able to do just that, you have to prioritize your nutritional needs. Even if you try to perform all kinds of exercises, you can't expect them to help you lose your overall weight or thigh fat if you do not follow healthy eating practices. Follow these steps to eating well in order to get slimmer thighs.

1. Go for nutritionally correct foods.

First thing on your list of things to do is to get proper nutrition. This is possible by eating nutritionally correct foods. The proper types of foods will help your body shed off excess weight from your entire body, including the fat in your thigh areas. Health experts recommend that you regularly eat any combination of the following foods and the like:

Vegetables: Broccoli, spinach, carrots and kale

Legumes: Beans, peas and lentils

Protein (lean): Fish, white poultry meat, dairy products and soy products

Grains (whole): Whole grain pasta

Fruits: Apples, pears, bananas, kiwi and citrus fruits

Seeds: Sunflower seeds, pumpkin seeds and flax seeds

Nuts: Walnuts and almonds

2. Make do with fewer carbohydrates.

To achieve your thigh fat loss goals, it is important that you eat less of carbohydrate-rich foods. When you consume more simple carbohydrates such as cookies, candies, and pasties, your metabolism gets affected in negative ways, which only cancel out the positive effect (and function) of carbohydrates – to provide your main energy source.

Look for ways to reduce your intake of carbohydrates like breads, pastas, and other forms of grains, which can cause you to feel less energetic as well as tire easily due to weight gain and decrease in blood sugar level. Choose to eat quinoa, brown rice, or other healthier grains instead of pasta or bread. Also, make it a point to replace baked goods, sugary desserts, and other artificially-sweetened food items with fresh fruits and other naturally sweet treats.

3. Up your protein intake.

Instead of eating pork or beef in order to increase your consumption of proteins, go for chicken, turkey, and other types of lean meat. Try to eat four servings of these healthy proteins every day, which is what is ideal for you (your fist equals one serving or about three to four ounces). Other sources of good protein are fish (best broiled or grilled) and eggs (best poached). It is essential for you to get the amount of energy you require (from proteins as well as grains), so you will have enough to perform your daily exercise routines and build muscle, especially in the thigh areas.

4. Cut down on sugar.

It is best to limit your intake of sugar as much as you can. Research has indicated that removing sugar from your diet helps in drastically lowering your overall calorie intake. To do just that, drink water (eight glasses daily) in place of any form of sugary drinks. You may also take green tea in place of sugary drinks. It contains beneficial antioxidants that can stimulate your metabolism.

Use honey, cinnamon and other natural sweeteners to add to your beverages. You may also use Stevia (derived from a plant in South America) as a sugar substitute in your coffee. It tastes just as sweet as sugar does, but without all that calories that sugar gives. Keep in mind that it is best to avoid all kinds of artificial sweeteners, and make sure that no corn syrup has been added to any of the food items you purchase by reading list of ingredients on their packages first. Avoid alcoholic beverages if you are serious about eating well, since these drinks contain high amounts of sugar.

5. Manage your calorie consumption.

It is important to monitor your intake of calories. Doing so will help you follow an improved diet plan as well as avoid improper eating habits. Consider your physical activity level and weight when computing your caloric requirements on a daily basis then make sure to record your daily calorie consumption for an entire month. You should also remember that besides ensuring your intake of healthy calories, it is also important that you control your blood sugar levels. This will help in making you feel satisfied and full after eating your meals as well as prevent food cravings.

6. Keep your blood sugar level steady.

Take note of any instances wherein you experience feeling cranky or tired between meals. You may observe that there are particular times in the day when your energy decreases. To combat lethargy, always carry around healthy snacks to prevent your blood sugar level from dipping. It also helps to forego eating any heavy carbohydrates, like bread, during lunch to avoid feeling sleepy by late afternoon.

It is also important that you take note of any food triggers you may have surrendered to, as well as any meals that are inappropriate for your healthy diet goals. You may find that you tend to eat cookies when you are stressed, or you always want to have some wine (a glass or two) whenever you are in the company of friends. Know that you should recognize whatever your triggers are so that you can effectively overcome them.

Instead of cookies, have a fruit. Instead of wine, have some green tea or water. A glass is recommended before eating your meals. Doing so helps kick start your metabolism while preventing you from overeating through suppression of your hunger.

7. Do away with the wrong kinds of food.

By all means, avoid all kinds of foods that cause your blood sugar level to spike (sodas and other sugary drinks, candies, cakes, and other forms of refined sugars), foods that contain trans fats or saturated fats (solid shortening, margarine, butter, and lard), foods that are overly processed (canned soups, frozen meals, deli meats, and breakfast cereals), as well as foods made of simple carbohydrates (white bread and regular pasta).

Enjoying the foods you eat as you try to eat healthily can help you control your weight, as well as get the energy you need to work out your thighs with strengthening and toning exercises. You will soon see the result of your effort to eat real foods over processed ones – thinner and better-looking thighs.

8. Practice proper hydration.

In case you choose to go on a healthy liquid diet, make sure that you hydrate your body without any unnecessary sweet additives. It is best to just stick to plain water to quench your thirst, as well as carry essential nutrients to your cells, flush out any harmful toxins out if your system, and lubricate your body tissues for their normal functioning. Health experts recommend drinking eight 8-oz. glasses of water per day.

Concentrated juices, sodas, and energy drinks only make losing overall fat, as well as fat in your thighs, difficult. You will be better off avoiding them. These drinks contain high amounts of sugar (up to 300 calories), negating any positive effects from an entire workout session. Try unsweetened green tea, which contains almost zero calories (at one to calories only per liter). Drinking one cup of green tea is also one way of tricking your body into feeling more full, which helps you eat less during meals.

9. Say no to eating more at night.

It pays to do more of your eating during mornings and less during evenings. It is important to eat a healthy breakfast anyway to ensure that you will have enough energy to kick your day off to a good start, as well as allow you to do your duties. The opposite applies to eating at night. Make sure that you eat less food in the evening, especially right before your bedtime. The reason for this is not a slower metabolism at night. It has something to do, instead, with the fact that you are more likely to eat poor snack choices during nighttime.

Chapter 2 - Work Out your Entire Body

It can take a while before you may be able to burn off the fat in and around your thighs. When you try to lose fat, your body naturally loses fat all over and not in a single area, such as your thighs. The best you can do is to have your body undergo workout routines that aim to make you lose overall fat and, as a result, make you lose the fat in your thighs as well. You will get the slim thighs you want. You just have to practice patience, do lots of walking, and perform resistance training.

Walk your Way to Thinner Thighs

Whenever and wherever you can, just walk. In fact, walk if you have nothing else to do. Walking may be the most underrated type of exercise there is, especially if you take into consideration the reality that it is able to burn away about 100 to 400 calories in an hour (depending on factors like your pace and weight).

You also have to take into account the fact that walking does not exhaust you as much as biking, running, or swimming does for the same amount of calories burned, making it an ideal form of thigh fat-losing exercise.

1. Keep it slow and steady.

It is essential to keep your walking pace risk and steady. A simple way to gauge if you are walking too fast is to check whether you can still carry on talking with a friend without getting breathless.

2. Practice good walking technique.

Make sure to keep your back straight while you are walking. Your toes should also point straight ahead. Walk with your head held up and your shoulders as well as chest lifted. You also have to ensure landing on your heels, after which you should push off from the toes as you roll forward on the balls of your feet. When walking up hills, or at a faster pace, make it a point to slightly lean forward.

3. Think about your safety and comfort.

It is also important to dress comfortably when planning to go for a walk. Go for lightweight clothing, which makes it easy to try dressing in layers. This makes it less difficult for you to cool yourself off, since you are just going to peel them off, layer by layer. Safety should also be your consideration when walking, so wear a reflective vest over your light-colored clothing. You will get noticed and be able to seek help faster that way. Also, it pays to walk in safe places (park trails, shopping malls, sidewalks on quiet streets, or your local school's athletic tracks).

4. Make sure to warm up first and cool down after.

Always warm up for five minutes before walking, and never miss doing a 5-minute cool down after each workout. When trying to warm up, make sure to start walking gradually. Meanwhile, it helps to do some stretching while you cool down.

5. Take it easy.

Go for long and easy strides to prevent straining yourself. If going faster is your aim, take longer strides instead of trying to walk at a faster pace.

6. Take care of your feet.

Wearing a pair of shoes that are good for your feet will go a long way if you want to stick to your walking routine. Buy a pair that comes with nylon mesh or other breathable upper material. Also, check to make sure that it cushions your feet with thick and flexible soles, and that your heels are elevated about ½-inch to ¾-inch above the soles.

7. Gently speed things up.

Allow both your arms to swing at the sides freely as you walk. This enables you to speed things up, especially if you bend both your elbows (an angle of 90 degrees works best for doing this).

Get Slimmer Thighs with Resistance Training

It is time to complement your walking exercises with resistance training routines after you notice that you have lost about one to two inches around your thighs. To help build up your muscles gradually, begin your resistance training on exercise machines using lighter weights and applying smaller amounts of resistance.

1. Pay more attention on form over weight.

Through all your exercise routines, make sure that your body is properly aligned and is moving in a smooth manner to avoid any injuries as well as to achieve faster results. A lot of experts agree that it would be better to learn a new routine in strength training if you use extremely light weights (or none at all) in the beginning. It also helps to focus on one muscle group as you smoothly perform gradual lifts and controlled falls.

2. Make it a regular thing.

It truly pays to exercise with strength training on a regular basis. Twice or thrice per week is the ideal number of times that will allow you to work all your body's major muscles.

3. Get warmed up and cooled down for more than two minutes.

Five to 10 minutes should be sufficient for a good warming up (such as walking) and cooling down (like stretching) session.

4. Give your muscles a challenge.

Constantly challenging your muscles will help a lot in giving you slimmer thighs. Opt to use weights that let you keep a good form while doing a routine, especially in the final two repetitions. Pick out an even lighter weight if doing the final 2 reps is difficult for you.

On the other hand, if completing all the reps no longer feels like a challenge, then it is time to push you to a higher level by adding heavier weights, doing more repetitions, or exercising for more than the usual two to three days per week. The important thing to keep in mind is that you should perform all repetitions and still maintain your good form while straining your targeted (thigh) muscles.

5. Don't forget to breathe.

Holding your breath during exercise can cause your blood pressure level to rise, so make sure that you breathe out as you perform different resistance training steps such as pulling, pushing, and lifting, and inhale upon release.

6. Know that tempo counts a lot in strength training.

Maintaining a tempo allows you to be in charge of your workout rather than letting momentum take its course and taking your strengthening benefits away.

7. Let your muscles rest.

It is essential that you allow your muscles to have some time off. Your muscle tissues can get slightly torn when you make them undergo strength training, which is the point of this type of exercise. As the tears in your muscles mend, those muscles will become stronger. Make sure to let two days pass before getting into another workout session to let your muscles recover.

Chapter 3 - Follow a Low-Fat, Low-Calorie Diet Plan

There is absolutely no way to justify starving yourself in order to lose the fat in your thighs. Keeping yourself from eating well only causes your metabolism to work at a slower rate, resulting in you having an unhealthy body as well as a difficult time losing any fat at all. It may be best for you to follow instead a healthy diet plan that reduces your overall fat and calorie intake in order to achieve your thigh fat loss goals.

1. Know the basics of the low-fat, low-calorie diet.

It is important that you know the nitty-gritty behind this diet plan. It works simply because it helps you reserve only enough calories in your body to burn off as well as help it function normally.

It also helps to understand that making the fat in your thighs go away is impossible, even with the best thought-out diet plan in the world. You need to decrease your total body fat in order to reduce your thigh fat, and the ideal way to do just that is to follow your diet and complement it with exercises that target your problem thighs.

2. Decrease the overall amount of calories you consume.

Reducing your overall intake of calories is key to losing the fat in your problem thighs. Women who perform moderate activities will do best lowering their daily calorie consumption to about 1200 calories to 1500 calories. Meanwhile, men who are also moderately active are advised to cut their calorie intake down to about 1500 calories to 1800 calories per day.

An extremely important thing to keep in mind is to never go below a mere 1000 calories per day (if you are a woman) or just 1200 calories daily (if you are a man). Other essential tips to follow daily include eating no more than 35 grams to 50 grams of fat, consuming about 170grams to 240 grams of carbohydrates, and getting anywhere from 55 grams to 95 grams of proteins.

3. Reduce your consumption of saturated fats.

You consume saturated fats when you eat foods containing hydrogenated oils, milk and dairy products, meats, and other animal sources. They make your food taste great but are in no way better compared to unsaturated fats, which you can usually get from plant sources.

Avoid coconut and palm oils because they are the sources of the highest saturated fat content, although butter as well as shortening, lard, and other rendered fats from animal sources also carry rich amounts of saturated fats. Meanwhile, even the healthy fish oil is bursting with saturated fats along with its omega-3 fatty acids.

It would also be best for you to avoid eating processed meats, cheese, seeds, nuts, dried coconut, and whipped cream, since they are all teeming with high amounts of saturated fat. The same goes for fast foods – you definitely can do without them. Keep in mind, however, that the message here is not to eliminate your consumption of saturated fats altogether. They still have health benefits that your body should take advantage of. Just make sure to limit your saturated fat intake to maximize their benefits.

4. Say no to anything that can cause your diet to go bust.

Granted, it would be unrealistic to think that you would be able to follow your low-fat, low-calorie diet plan to the letter at all times, but it would be best for you to avoid eating anything, even in small amounts, that can make you decide to quit your diet. These foods include prepackaged snacks, boxed meals that are available at the grocery store, greasy food found in restaurants, and any kind of processed foods, especially those made with hydrogenated oils. Also, avoid drinking alcohol. They do contain high amounts of calories that only add to your problem with your fat thighs.

5. Do away with red meat.

It is far better to eat lean protein instead of red meat, since the former has lower amounts of saturated fats as well as less amounts of calories. Instead of pork and beef, go for turkey, chicken, and fish that you should eat fresh. You can also use lentils, pinto beans, and other legumes to replace red meat in your diet.

6. Eat lots of dairy that are low in fat.

Dairy can be fattening, but it contains calcium, which is also good for your body, so it is not sensible to eliminate it completely from your diet. To benefit from milk without its fattening tendencies, select low-fat variants over whole and use cottage cheese and yogurt instead of butters and creams.

7. Think whole grains.

Complex carbohydrates like whole grains help your body lose overall fat as well as thigh fat because they require more energy from your body to burn them off. To get the most out of the whole grains' ability to help trim your thighs, avoid any food item made with processed flour and go instead for crackers, cereals, breads, and other grain products that are baked using oats, whole wheat, and other forms of whole grain. Also, consume more of vegetables and fruits because they are rich in complex carbohydrates as well.

Chapter 4 - Target your Thighs

It's unrealistic to think you can lose your thigh fat with only a couple of exercise routines. You can only expect to see tangible results within one month to six weeks, especially if you are targeting your thighs about thrice a week. You don't even have to use any complicated exercise machine – just follow these thigh-targeting moves.

I. Do the towel squeeze.

1. With your knees on a bending position, put your back in a lying-down position on the floor. Keep your feet flat on their soles and your arms flat and relaxed on either side while fixing your gaze straight ahead.

2. Insert a small folded towel between your left and right knees.

3. Keeping your knees close to each other, squeeze them into the inserted towel. Raise your hips as high as possible. Lower your hips after holding for two counts, and then do 15 repetitions.

II. Squat and pick up dumbbells.

1. Position your feet away from each other at a shoulder-wide distance while letting each of your hand hold an eight-pound dumbbell by the side.

2. Get your knees to bend at an angle of 90 degrees. Put down each dumbbell outside your left and right foot while making sure your chest is lifted.

3. Get yourself to a standing position and then back to a squatting position as you pick up the weights again.

4. Do the same routine for one minute; alternate picking up and lowering of the weights.

III. Make like a frog.

1. Lay your arms by your sides in a relaxing way as you place your back on the mat or ground.

2. Draw in your abdomen as you gradually tuck your knees in, chest-wards.

3. Do flexing motions with each of your left and right foot while bending your knees outwards and sideward. Make sure your heels are touching each other.

4. Move your legs with a pressing motion to widen them at an angle of 45 degrees, and then bring together your inner thighs by squeezing your knees' backs close to one another.

5. Keeping the same angle of 45 degrees, bend your knees in again.

6. Do the same movement in 15 repetitions.

IV. Do some plyometric squatting.

1. Place your two feet apart from each other at a shoulder-wide distance.

2. Bring your body down to a squatting position as you bend your knees at an angle of 90 degrees.

3. Bring your body to a standing position by jumping up (using your legs' and butt's strengths), and then get back into your

squatting position by landing softly on the ground.

4. Softly land again on the ground to a squatting position, keeping your knees bent this time and your weight back.

5. Do three sets of the same routine in 8 repetitions.

V. Kick around and stretch out.

1. Hold onto a chair's back while standing and pressing your shoulder blades backwards and downwards.

2. Raise your right leg after bringing your weight onto your left foot's ball part.

3. Pull your abdominal muscles in and lift your right leg over your left leg across your torso.

4. Swing your right leg out to your right side while maintaining the position of your flexed toes and turned-out toes. Let momentum do the work of swinging your right leg through the left part of your butt.

5. Keeping your hips in a face-forward position, do 10 repetitions of this movement to complete a set.

6. Do the same routine with your left leg.

7. Perform a second set after taking a breather.

VI. Make like a skater.

1. Bring your feet together with the toes pointed in a forward direction. Place each of your arms by your left and right side, and keep your head and neck facing straight ahead.

2. Using your right foot, do a wide-skate step to your right side. Bring your left foot toward your right foot in a dragging motion while allowing your left arm to reach forward. Bring your right elbow in again to do a skating motion.

3. As fast as you can manage, change directions and do the same movement using your left foot.

4. Perform as many repetitions as you possibly can in one minute, doing alternate movements from the left side to the left side.

VII. Do a lying-down circle tracing.

1. Lie down with your back on the mat, making sure that your arms are by your left and right side and that your palms are placed face-down on the mat.

2. Using your toes, point your left foot upward and then slightly rotate your leg outward.

3. Breathe in as you use your left leg to trace on the ceiling a circular shape. Move your entire leg while preventing your left hip from being lifted off the mat.

4. Moving your leg clockwise, do the same tracing movement in 5 repetitions. Do the same movement in the opposite direction (counter-clockwise).

5. Do the same routine on your right leg in 5 repetitions.

VIII. Sit on your heels with a ball.

1. Insert a ball between the area where your lower back curves and the wall.

2. Stand straight as you position your feet apart with a shoulder-wide distance between them.

3. Get your knees to a bending position and, making sure your hips are square and your shoulders are level, lower your body about five to ten inches. Return to a standing position after holding the bending pose for about three seconds.

4. Do 5 repetitions of this exercise before moving up to twelve, making sure to rest for half a minute before doing another set.

IX. Work your inner thigh area.

1. Using your left leg, do a standing position. Raise your right leg above the ground by a couple of inches while bending your knee.

2. Twist your left knee sideways, and then raise your right heel above your head while bringing your left leg across your body at the front.

3. Bring your right leg down, and then raise it up while keeping your heel up as well.

4. Do 15 repetitions of this exercise on each side.

X. Perform seated knee bends.

1. Press your hands on the floor while sitting down, with your hands placed on either side of your hips.

2. Bring your knees to an inward bending position. Let your knees touch and hold that position as you point your toes and you fix your gaze straight ahead.

3. Contract your muscles in the abdomen as you slightly lean forward.

4. Keep your knees opened to either side as you trace the floor with your toes, and then bring your knees together so that they touch.

5. Do 20 repetitions of this movement.

XI. Greet the sun.

1. Stand tall on your exercise mat. Make sure your feet are close together, your arms are by

left and right sides, and your weight is evenly distributed through your soles.

2. Do a single deep breath as you lift your two arms above your head while slightly raising your chin. Use your fingertips to reach toward the direction of the sky as you keep your palms facing one another and your arms straightened out.

3. From the second step, bring your arms to your sides with a sweeping-down motion. Make sure to breathe out as you do a forward swan-dive as you bend forward. Bend your body at the hips as you try to touch the mat on the sides of your two feet with your fingertips or palms. If you feel like any area around your hamstrings or back start to tighten, try bending your knees while keeping your fingers in perfect alignment with your toes.

4. From the third step, place your back flat on the mat, and then breathe in as you lift your torso to your waist height while maintaining your back's flat position. Fix your eyes toward your front while you reach with your behind away from your head's crown. Make sure that your head is in alignment with your backbone and that your navel is pulled in.

5. Bend your body at the knees and then position your palms flat and face-down on the mat, keeping a shoulder-wide distance between them.

6. Walk backwards and then lift your pelvis (hips) until you assume a downward-facing dog position. Keep your fingers spread out and your feet parallel and apart with a hip-wide distance between them. Do a reaching pose with your behind facing the sky and hold the position for several seconds as you breathe.

Conclusion

Thank you again for purchasing this book!

I hope this book was able to help you to get even more inspired to trimming off the unhealthy and unwanted fats in your thighs right now. You only need to follow everything that is presented in this book in order to make your thigh fat loss dream possible.

The next step is to be realistic when it comes to trying to change how your body and especially your thighs appear. So what if they touch? That is only normal for men and women alike. Your goal should be to make your thighs look leaner so that you will feel more comfortable in your clothes, and so that you will feel more at ease doing your daily tasks (you can now say goodbye to chafing!). Accept your thighs for the best that they can be, not for what they should look like.

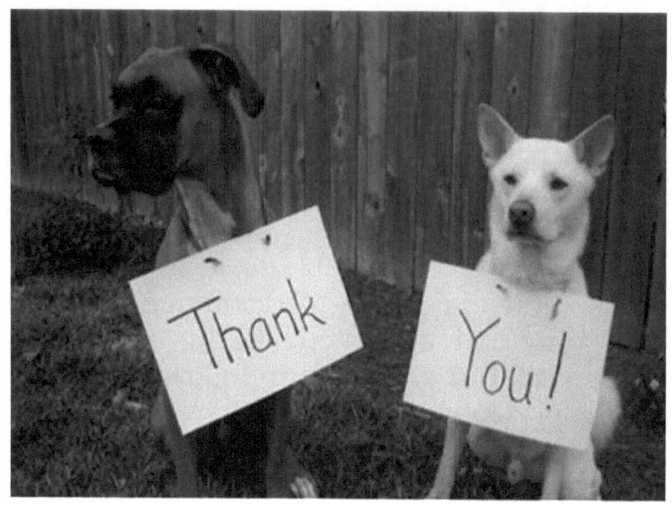

Finally, if you enjoyed this book, then I'd like to ask you for a favor, would you be kind enough to leave a review for this book on Amazon? It'd be greatly appreciated!

Thank you and good luck!

BONUS: FREE Books for You

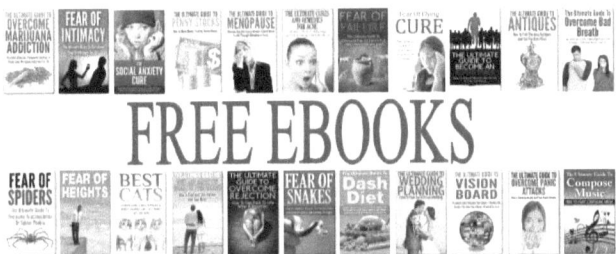

Dear reader!

If you like my books, I'd like to share more books with you FOR FREE.

When I place my book for free promotion, and the cost of the books is $ 0.00, I can send you the link for free download, and you can save up to $ 10 every time.

Simply copy this link and paste it to your browser – http://bit.ly/1MD7sXu

Check Out My Other Books

Below you'll find some of my other popular books that are popular on Amazon and Kindle as well. Simply click on the links below to check them out. Alternatively, you can visit my author page on Amazon to see other work done by me. If the links do not work, for whatever reason, you can simply search for these titles on the Amazon website to find them.

1) The Ultimate Guide To CheerLeading - How To Become A Pro Cheerleader And Start To Win Everywhere

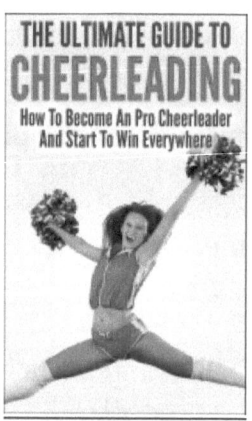

Or go to: http://amzn.to/1HZCdJJ

2) The Ultimate Guide To Become An Alpha Female - How To Attract Men, Win In Life And Be Confident

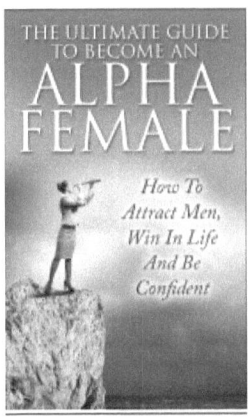

Or go to: http://amzn.to/1NFrQHv

Thanks You!

Allison Lewis